The Acid Reflux Solution

A Comprehensive Guide to Naturally Preventing and Managing Gastroesophageal Reflux Disease (GERD) and Its Symptoms

Isabella White

Disclaimer: *The information in this book is based on the author's research, opinions, and experiences. It is not intended to replace professional medical advice or treatment. The reader should regularly consult a physician for any health issues and always seek the advice of a physician before modifying diet, supplement, or exercise regimens. The author and publisher shall have neither liability nor responsibility to any person or entity concerning any loss or damage related to the information contained in this book. The information provided is general and may not apply to every individual. Any reliance on the information contained herein is solely at the reader's risk.*

Table of Contents

Appendices_____ **63**

Introduction

Gastroesophageal reflux disease, commonly called GERD, occurs when stomach acid frequently flows back up into the esophagus. This backflow of acid is called acid reflux. The esophagus is the tube that carries food and liquids from your mouth down to your stomach. At the lower end of the esophagus is a ring-like muscle known as the lower esophageal sphincter, or LES.

Normally, the LES closes tightly after food passes through to the stomach. However, when the LES relaxes inappropriately or weakens, acidic stomach contents can regurgitate up into the esophagus, causing irritation and pain.

Acid reflux causes a burning sensation in the chest, known as heartburn. Other common symptoms include a sour or bitter taste in the mouth, excessive burping, chest pain, chronic sore throat, laryngitis, and difficulty swallowing. Prolonged exposure of the esophagus to corrosive stomach acid can lead to more dangerous complications such as esophagitis, strictures, Barrett's esophagus, and, in rare cases, esophageal cancer. GERD symptoms negatively impact the quality of life and the enjoyment of meals.

GERD affects over 60 million Americans to some degree. Obesity, pregnancy, certain medications, and a hiatal hernia can increase the risk of developing GERD. Hiatal hernias occur when part of the stomach bulges up into the chest through an opening in the diaphragm.

Factors like diet, excess weight, smoking, and alcohol use also contribute to a weak LES. Stress aggravates hyperacidity and is linked to more severe GERD. Even perfectly healthy individuals can experience occasional reflux when they overeat, exercise right after meals, or lay down before properly digesting food.

The good news is that GERD can be effectively controlled and prevented through diet, lifestyle changes, stress management, and natural remedies. With the comprehensive information in this book, you will better understand the underlying causes of your acid reflux. Armed with this knowledge and positive habits, you can break your dependence on antacids and acid blockers to achieve lasting freedom from GERD symptoms.

The Prevalence and Impact of GERD on Daily Life

Acid reflux is a widespread problem, affecting millions of Americans. Approximately 20% of the adult population experiences acid reflux symptoms at least once a week. The prevalence of GERD has increased dramatically in recent decades. Several factors contribute to this, including rising obesity rates, an aging population, and increased awareness and diagnosis. It is estimated that 60% of asthma patients also suffer from GERD, hinting at a correlation between the two conditions.

Frequent acid reflux takes a tangible toll on people's health and quality of life. The painful burning sensation of heartburn can interrupt sleep, reduce work productivity, and limit enjoyment of meals. 75% of people with nighttime GERD symptoms say it negatively impacts their sleep quality. Sleep deprivation then exacerbates acid reflux symptoms, creating a vicious cycle. The constant discomfort and distress of chronic GERD can lead to increased anxiety and depression.

Acid reflux symptoms strike during holidays and social gatherings centered around food and drinks. This can cause embarrassment and discourage sufferers from fully participating. They may avoid favorite foods and beverages that trigger flare-ups, such as citrus, tomato sauce, coffee, and alcohol. GERD dietary restrictions also hamper the spontaneity of eating out and traveling.

Long-term acid exposure in the esophagus alters cell structure, increasing cancer risk. Esophageal cancer rates have increased by over 500% in the last four decades. Once diagnosed, the 5-year survival rate is only about 20%. Managing GERD early and effectively is imperative.

The good news is that, in many cases, you have the power to prevent and treat acid reflux through diet and lifestyle changes alone. With the comprehensive guidance provided in this book, you can avoid medications and enjoy freedom from GERD and its detrimental effects. Simple natural remedies can quickly provide relief when symptoms flare up. You will reclaim confidence in social situations and the quality of life you deserve.

Importance of Natural Prevention and Management

Conventional treatment for acid reflux typically involves antacids and medications like proton pump inhibitors (PPIs) or H2 blockers. These medications only provide temporary relief and do not address the underlying causes of reflux. Long-term use can lead to side effects, nutritional deficiencies, and increased vulnerability to infections. Natural solutions are the optimal approach for preventing and managing acid reflux.

Lifestyle factors play a huge role in causing and controlling GERD. Dietary triggers, lack of exercise, smoking, and stress are major contributing factors to acid reflux. By making simple but consistent changes in these areas, many find they can resolve symptoms and avoid medications. Diet and lifestyle modifications should be the first line of defense against GERD.

Additionally, many natural remedies provide quick and effective symptom relief during flare-ups. Chewing gum, aloe vera juice, baking soda water, and herbal teas are some simple solutions that can quickly calm reflux. Essential oils like peppermint and ginger also relax the digestive tract. Identifying go-to natural alternatives empowers sufferers to self-treat symptoms when they strike.

Weaning off antacids and acid blockers requires gradually reducing dependence while implementing lifestyle changes to address the root causes. With dedication and patience, you can break the cycle of acid-suppressing medications. The natural prevention techniques and solutions outlined in this book allow you to take control of your health and achieve drug-free acid reflux management.

Promoting gut health with probiotic foods and supplements reduces long-term reflux. Probiotics balance the bacteria in your digestive system to optimize functioning. Stress management and natural remedies that improve esophageal function strengthen your defenses against GERD.

The natural world provides us with safe, affordable tools to prevent and treat acid reflux effectively if we take the time to make the necessary lifestyle changes. By avoiding triggers, reducing pressure on the LES, and utilizing natural remedies during flare-ups, you can get lasting relief without dependence on medications. Arm yourself with the knowledge and positive habits outlined in this book to prevent and manage GERD for good naturally.

Chapter 1

Understanding Acid Reflux and GERD

What Happens in the Body to Cause Acid Reflux?

Acid reflux is a digestive disorder that occurs when stomach acid and other contents flow back into the esophagus. This happens when the lower esophageal sphincter (LES) weakens or inappropriately relaxes. The LES is a circular muscle band located at the point where the esophagus and stomach meet.

Normally, the LES remains tightly closed to function as a valve that allows food to pass into the stomach but prevents stomach acid from escaping back into the esophagus.

However, acid can reflux into the esophagus when this valve mechanism is impaired, causing burning discomfort. There are a few ways the LES can become compromised.

First, the LES may relax temporarily from normal triggers like heavy meals, alcohol, chocolate, or coffee. When the stomach is full, pressure builds up, forcing the LES to open. The LES then closes again normally after belching or vomiting relieves the pressure.

Frequent heavy meals and portion sizes stretch the stomach over time, causing the LES to lose tone and weaken. Obesity also increases pressure on the LES.

A hiatal hernia can interfere with LES function. This occurs when the upper part of the stomach protrudes through the diaphragm into the chest cavity. Hiatal hernias prevent the LES from closing securely. About 50% of GERD patients have a hiatal hernia.

Hormones may play a role as well. Pregnancy can cause acid reflux due to hormonal changes that soften the LES. Heightened stress levels also increase stomach acid production while simultaneously relaxing the LES.

Certain medications can contribute to a weakened LES by irritating the esophageal lining or relaxing the LES, including NSAIDs, calcium channel blockers, sedatives, antidepressants, and opioids. Smoking also lowers LES pressure and provokes coughing fits that can trigger reflux.

Understanding how the LES malfunctions provides clear ways to prevent and minimize acid reflux. Losing excess weight, eating smaller meals, avoiding dietary triggers, managing stress, and quitting smoking can all help maintain a properly functioning LES.

Risk Factors and Causes of Acid Reflux

A variety of factors can increase susceptibility to acid reflux. The most common risk factors and causes include:

1. **Diet:** Foods that weaken or put pressure on the LES provoke reflux. Common triggers are fatty foods, chocolate, onions, citrus fruit, tomatoes, coffee, alcohol, and mint. Large, heavy meals also overload the stomach. Eating late at night means food sits in the stomach longer while lying down.

2. **Obesity:** Excess weight strains the LES and increases pressure on the stomach. Fat around the abdomen pushes on the stomach, forcing contents upwards. Obesity increases reflux symptoms by 2–3

fold. Losing weight improves symptoms dramatically.

3. **Pregnancy:** Hormonal changes and abdominal pressure from the growing fetus cause acid reflux in up to 80% of pregnant women. Symptoms typically resolve after giving birth.

4. **Hiatal hernia:** When part of the stomach pushes through the diaphragm into the chest, it obstructs the LES valve mechanism. About 60% of GERD patients have a hiatal hernia.

5. **Smoking:** Nicotine weakens the LES and stimulates acid production. Chronic coughing from smoking also triggers reflux. Quitting provides major relief.

6. **Certain medications:** Drugs that relax the LES or irritate the esophagus provoke reflux. These include anticholinergics, calcium channel blockers, sedatives, NSAIDs, and opioids.

7. **Stress and anxiety:** Stress hormones increase stomach acid production while relaxing the LES. Managing stress levels prevents flare-ups.

8. **Structural issues:** Conditions such as tumors, strictures, or spasms in the esophagus can obstruct stomach emptying and cause reflux.

9. **Insufficient digestive enzymes:** Inadequate levels of enzymes compromise digestion, causing undigested food to ferment and produce gases that force open the LES.

10. **Age:** The LES weakens and loses tone naturally with age, increasing elderly reflux risk. Acid secretion also declines with age.

11. **Family history:** Up to 25% of GERD patients have a first-degree relative with the condition. Genetics may play a role in LES dysfunction.

Identifying specific triggers and risk factors allows you to effectively minimize episodes through preventative lifestyle measures and natural acid reflux remedies.

The Common Symptoms

Acid reflux can cause various symptoms, ranging from mild to severe. Recognizing the signs of reflux is key to getting an accurate diagnosis and formulating an effective treatment plan. Here are some of the most common symptoms associated with acid reflux:

1. **Heartburn:** A burning pain in the chest or throat after eating is heartburn. The lining of the esophagus becomes irritated due to stomach acid.

2. **Regurgitation:** A perception of food or sour-tasting acid backing up into the throat or mouth, often accompanied by a "wet burp." This occurs when the stomach contents are regurgitated into the esophagus.

3. **Dysphagia:** Difficulty swallowing or the sensation of food getting stuck. Chronic acid irritation causes inflammation and strictures or narrowing of the esophagus.

4. **Chronic sore throat:** Frequent coughing, hoarseness, or sore throat can indicate acid reflux is impacting the throat and vocal cords. This is known as LPR (laryngopharyngeal reflux).

5. **Excessive burping:** Constant belching or burping after meals increases stomach gas with the acid, worsening reflux. This removes pressure on the LES but causes painful gas reflux.

6. **Chest pain:** A heavy, squeezing sensation or dull ache in the chest may mimic heart attack symptoms. Acid reflux causes painful esophageal spasms.

7. **Bad breath:** When refluxed liquid sits in the esophagus or mouth, bacteria feed on it and release gases, causing halitosis or bad breath.

8. **Eroded tooth enamel:** Chronic exposure to stomach acid can damage tooth enamel and lead to decay and sensitivity.

9. **Chronic cough:** Acid irritation produces coughing spells or wheezing in some GERD patients, especially at night or after meals.

10. **Disrupted sleep:** Nocturnal reflux and chest discomfort make it difficult to sleep. Insomnia can further exacerbate acid reflux symptoms.

11. **Nausea:** The urge to vomit, especially after meals, may signal excess stomach acid production, which is irritating.

Paying close attention to symptoms and when they occur provides you and your doctor with key insights for developing an optimal treatment strategy. Keeping a symptom journal is recommended to identify reflux triggers.

Consequences of Acid Reflux Left Untreated

While occasional acid reflux is normal, chronic exposure to stomach acid can inflict serious damage if left untreated. Some consequences of uncontrolled GERD include:

1. **Esophagitis:** Stomach acid erodes, inflames, and damages the lining of the esophagus. This can cause bleeding, pain with swallowing, and ulcers. Esophagitis also leads to Barrett's esophagus.

2. **Strictures:** Chronic inflammation and scarring cause narrowing and stiffness of the esophagus. Strictures obstruct swallowing. Foods get stuck, causing pain and vomiting.

3. **Barrett's esophagus:** Precancerous intestinal-like cells replace damaged esophageal lining cells from repeated acid exposure. This disorder increases esophageal cancer risk substantially.

4. **Esophageal ulcers:** Painful open sores called peptic ulcers form in the lining when eroded. Ulcers bleed easily and are slow to heal.

5. **Pneumonia and asthma:** When stomach contents are aspirated into the lungs, it can lead to pneumonia, bronchitis, and wheezing and aggravate asthma.

6. **Eroded tooth enamel:** Stomach acid contacting teeth frequently over time erodes tooth enamel and causes decay more easily.

7. **Recurrent sinus and ear infections:** Postnasal drip from GERD carries acid into nasal and ear

passages, resulting in chronic congestion and infections.

8. **Laryngitis:** Acid larynx irritation causes chronic hoarseness, coughing, and difficulty speaking. Frequent throat clearing is common.

9. **Iron and vitamin B12 deficiency:** Impaired absorption of critical nutrients due to damaged stomach and esophageal cells leads to anemia.

10. **Sleep apnea:** Acid reflux worsens sleep apnea. The use of CPAP machines can provoke nighttime reflux in turn.

Prolonged acid reflux without treatment compromises your health and quality of life substantially, in addition to increasing your cancer risk. Implementing this book's prevention and treatment strategies enables you to avoid these harmful consequences. Do not resign to living with acid reflux; take control of your health starting today.

Difference Between Acid Reflux and GERD

Acid reflux refers to the backward flow of stomach acid into the esophagus. It is very common, occurring in most people occasionally. About 60% of the population experiences acid reflux at least once a month.

In contrast, GERD (gastroesophageal reflux disease) refers specifically to reflux that occurs frequently enough to negatively impact quality of life or cause complications like esophagitis and Barrett's esophagus. GERD is a chronic, more severe form of acid reflux.

The difference lies primarily in the frequency and severity of symptoms. Occasional heartburn after large meals does not mean you have GERD. Everyone experiences benign reflux now and then when eating certain trigger foods or overeating. However, consistent reflux symptoms that disrupt sleep and daily living indicate GERD.

While acid reflux may cause only temporary discomfort, GERD manifests as severe heartburn and regurgitation at least twice a week or even daily. Symptoms are severe enough to undermine quality of life and require medical intervention. Damage may occur in the lining of the esophagus. Other extra-esophageal symptoms like hoarseness, wheezing, or coughing fit the criteria for GERD.

Diagnosis also helps distinguish between acid reflux and GERD. Doctors rely on symptom frequency and an endoscopic exam of the esophagus. They look for signs of inflammation, ulcers, strictures, or precancerous cell changes indicative of GERD. A pH test monitoring esophageal acidity helps confirm a GERD diagnosis as well.

It is important to note that GERD is a progressive condition. Occasional acid reflux, if left untreated, can develop into more frequent, severe GERD over time as the esophagus becomes more damaged. Implementing lifestyle changes is critical to halting this progression.

The good news is that over 95% of chronic GERD cases can be successfully managed with diet, behavior modifications, stress relief, and natural remedies—the techniques you will learn in this book. While GERD implies a more serious, persistent condition, you can control symptoms and avoid complications through natural prevention.

Chapter 2

Lifestyle Modifications for Prevention and Symptom Management

Dietary Changes for Preventing and Managing Acid Reflux

Diet plays a huge role in controlling acid reflux symptoms. While certain foods and eating habits trigger reflux, others can help calm symptoms and strengthen your defenses against GERD. Some key dietary tips include:

- **Avoid known reflux triggers.** These common culprits worsen reflux by irritating the esophagus, weakening the LES, or increasing stomach acid. They include coffee, alcohol, chocolate, fried foods, citrus fruits, tomatoes, carbonated beverages, peppermint, garlic, and onions.

- **Eat smaller, more frequent meals.** Large portions overload the stomach, increasing pressure on the LES. Eating smaller portions 5–6 times daily gives the stomach less work. Do not lie down right after large meals.

- **Limit high-fat foods.** Fatty and fried foods sit longer in the stomach, and obesity stresses the LES. Choose lean proteins like chicken, fish, beans, and tofu.

- **Incorporate reflux-soothing foods.** Almond milk, oatmeal, broth-based soups, melon, ginger, fennel, and leafy greens help reduce stomach acid. Fresh pineapple contains bromelain to aid digestion.

- **Choose non-acidic foods.** Reflux-safe foods include rice, couscous, carrots, winter squash, collard greens, basil, and cucumbers. Acidic produce like berries, tomatoes, and citrus fruit can provoke symptoms.

- **Avoid trigger foods before bed.** Eating a large meal before lying down ensures that stomach contents reflux upward. Finish eating 3 hours before bedtime. Sleep with the head elevated if nighttime reflux is an issue.

- **Chew thoroughly.** Wolfing down food introduces more air, increasing stomach pressure. Chew each bite 20–30 times to aid digestion and make food easier on the LES.

- **Stay hydrated.** It is recommended to drink at least eight glasses of non-carbonated fluids daily and avoid alcohol and coffee. This can reduce pressure on the LES. Herbal tea and aloe vera juice can aid in healing tissues.

Most acid reflux sufferers find significant symptom relief and prevention with simple dietary adjustments. This allows you to avoid antacids and other medications for the long term.

Tips for Losing Weight to Help Prevent and Manage Acid Reflux

Excess weight significantly aggravates acid reflux in several ways. Abdominal fat puts physical pressure on the stomach, forcing contents into the esophagus. Obesity also causes the LES valve to weaken and lose tone over time. Losing 10–15 pounds can dramatically alleviate reflux symptoms in overweight individuals. Here are some tips to shed pounds safely:

- **Start a food diary.** Monitoring everything you eat helps identify problem areas like mindless snacking or excess calories from condiments and cooking oils.

- **Cut out sugary drinks.** Sodas, fruit juices, and specialty coffee drinks add empty calories. Stick to water, unsweetened tea, and coffee.

- **Watch portion sizes.** Use smaller plates and bowls to avoid dishing up too much food. Eat slowly and stop when you feel 80% full.

- **Choose lean proteins.** Stick to healthy, low-fat proteins like chicken, fish, eggs, beans, tofu, or Greek yogurt instead of red meat. Avoid fried options.

- **Fill up on non-starchy veggies.** Enjoy unlimited raw, roasted, or steamed vegetables to feel satisfied without consuming carbs and calories.

- **Reduce alcohol intake.** Alcohol is high in empty calories. Limit yourself to 1-2 drinks per week. Avoid mixed cocktails loaded with sugar.

- **Snack smart.** Swap out chips, cookies, and candy for fresh fruit, veggies with hummus, unsalted nuts, or popcorn.
- **Exercise regularly.** Aim for 30-45 minutes of brisk activity daily. Mix up cardio and strength training.
- **Get enough sleep.** Lack of sleep disrupts metabolism by regulating hormones, leading to weight gain. Aim for 7-9 hours a night.

With persistence and commitment to these lifestyle changes, you can achieve a healthier weight and significant relief from acid reflux. Every pound shed lessens the pressure contributing to your symptoms.

The Importance of Avoiding Food Right Before Bedtime

Eating a full meal shortly before going to bed is one of the worst habits when it comes to controlling acid reflux. Lying down right after eating ensures gravity no longer aids digestion, making reflux much more likely. Here is why you should avoid food 2-3 hours before bed:

When you eat a meal and lie flat, stomach contents press against a relaxed lower esophageal sphincter (LES). This allows acid to reflux easily into the esophagus, causing painful heartburn that can disrupt sleep. Remaining upright keeps gravity working in your favor to limit reflux.

Large meals fill and expand the stomach, increasing pressure on the LES. Overfilled stomachs take longer to fully empty. Lying down hampers digestion and emptying even more. It is best to stop eating when your stomach feels about 70% full to avoid overfilling.

Certain triggers can cause the Lower Esophageal Sphincter (LES) to relax, leading to increased production of stomach acid. This can be a cause of concern for many people. Common dietary triggers include tomatoes, citrus, chocolate, alcohol, peppermint, coffee, and fat. Consuming them in the evening is especially problematic because you remain horizontal before digestion completes.

When awake after a meal, you can physically relieve pressure on the LES by standing, walking, or sitting upright. Belching and passing gas also provide some relief. However, when sleeping, there is no chance for these pressure-relieving activities.

Nighttime heartburn disrupts restorative REM sleep. Tossing and turning from reflux pain leads to fatigue and impaired focus the next day. Lack of quality sleep then further aggravates acid reflux symptoms, fueling a vicious cycle.

Allowing undigested food and stomach acids to pool in the esophagus all night worsens damage to the esophageal lining. Over time, this increases your risk of complications like esophagitis, strictures, and Barrett's esophagus.

The 3-hour rule allows your main evening meal to fully digest before retiring to bed. For some, even more than 3 hours is required. Pay attention to your body's signals and allow at least 2 hours for digestion. Avoid snacks or drinks other than water after dinner as well.

Making this one lifestyle change can significantly alleviate nighttime reflux. Follow the 3-hour rule for lying down after eating to prevent undigested food from exerting pressure on your LES sphincter as you sleep.

Quitting Smoking and Limiting Alcohol Intake to Prevent Acid Reflux

Both tobacco smoking and excess alcohol strongly provoke acid reflux symptoms. Quitting smoking and restricting alcohol provides tremendous relief for many reflux sufferers. Here is how these habits aggravate reflux:

Smoking weakens and relaxes the lower esophageal sphincter (LES). This allows stomach contents to backwash into the esophagus. Smoking also stimulates the production of stomach acid while slowing digestion.

The nicotine and other chemicals in cigarettes directly irritate the esophageal lining, making it more sensitive to acid erosion. Chronic coughing from smoking also triggers reflux episodes by increasing abdominal pressure.

Smokers experience twice as many reflux episodes as non-smokers. Symptoms like heartburn, regurgitation, hoarseness, and wheezing are more frequent and severe in smokers. Quitting smoking is the #1 lifestyle change GERD patients can make.

Like smoking, alcohol is a prime instigator of acid reflux. All types of alcohol relax the LES, allowing acidic stomach juices to rise into the esophagus. Wine, beer, and liquor are all frequent culprits.

Alcohol also increases gastric acid production at the same time that it relaxes the LES. This combo leads to corrosive acid that can freely reflux into the esophagus when drinking.

Carbonated drinks like beer and champagne ferment in the stomach, releasing gases that pressure the LES. Cocktails with citrus, soda, or juice increase stomach acidity as well.

For those battling GERD, it is best to avoid alcohol completely. If abstaining proves difficult, restrict intake to one 5-ounce glass of wine or beer maximum, no more than twice weekly with a meal. Avoid liquor and mixed drinks.

Quitting smoking allows the esophagus to heal and strengthen against acid erosion over time. Cutting out alcohol provides immediate relief by eliminating a prime instigator of reflux episodes. Both steps are critical for preventing GERD complications.

Wearing Loose and Comfortable Clothing Can Help Prevent and Manage Acid Reflux

Tight, restrictive clothing exacerbates acid reflux symptoms in several ways. Wearing loose, comfortable garments can dramatically reduce pressure and discomfort. Here is how:

Tight pants, belts, shapewear, or slim-cut dresses apply external pressure to the abdomen. This physically squeezes the stomach, promoting the backwash of acidic contents into the esophagus.

Snug waistbands drive stomach contents upwards against a relaxed lower esophageal sphincter (LES). Gravity no longer aids digestion when contents are pushed higher than the stomach outlet.

Binding clothes limits your ability to relax and breathe deeply and fully. Shallow breathing reduces oxygenation, which is essential for proper digestion. Deep belly breathing also helps relieve pressure on the LES.

After eating large meals, tight clothes feel extra uncomfortable. You may unbutton pants or loosen belts for relief. Choose stretchy, loose styles that do not bind even with a full stomach.

For women, underwire bras can apply stomach-compressing pressure. Opt for soft, wireless bras without restrictive bands. Breathable natural fabrics like cotton and linen are best.

Look for pants with an elastic, adjustable waist or waistband-free silhouette. Yoga pants, knit skirts, maxi dresses, and flowy tops allow comfortable digestion.

Aim for a streamlined fit versus a skin-tight fit. You want clothes that gently skim your figure without clinging or squeezing. Proper circulation is important.

In addition to preventing reflux episodes, loose clothing allows you to relax and breathe easier. This helps reduce overall stress levels that compound digestive issues.

Wardrobe adjustments may seem minor, but they can make a surprising difference in reducing acid reflux flare-ups. Carefully consider fit and fabrics to relieve pressure on your stomach.

Chapter 3

Home Remedies and Natural Treatments

Natural Remedies for Treating Acid Reflux

In addition to diet and lifestyle changes, many natural home remedies provide quick relief from occasional acid reflux symptoms. Common options include:

1. **Baking soda:** A teaspoon of baking soda dissolved in water immediately neutralizes stomach acid. The alkaline solution calms inflammation and relieves painful burning. Stir 1/2 teaspoon into 4 ounces of water and drink slowly.

2. **Aloe vera juice:** The mucopolysaccharides in aloe vera help coat and soothe irritated esophageal tissue. Aloe vera also aids digestion. Drink 2 ounces 20 minutes before meals. Choose brands that are certified safe for internal use.

3. **Apple cider vinegar:** Counterintuitively, a small dose of acidic ACV boosts the stomach's acidic environment to prevent reflux. Mix 1-2 teaspoons in water and drink before heavy meals.

4. **Ginger:** Ginger root tea or candies provide fast relief by reducing spasms and gas production in the stomach after meals. Ginger also has anti-inflammatory properties.

5. **Fennel tea:** The anise flavor of fennel seeds has antispasmodic effects that relax smooth muscle tissue along the digestive tract, reducing acid reflux after meals.

6. **Licorice root:** Licorice root increases the mucus coating of esophageal tissues, providing a protective barrier against stomach acid erosion. Limit intake to avoid side effects.

7. **Slippery elm:** The mucilage in slippery elm bark coats, soothes, and protects against acid burn. Enjoy as a tea or lozenge.

These remedies work best for occasional mild symptoms rather than severe, chronic GERD cases. They provide quick relief in combination with dietary and preventative lifestyle changes. Discuss incorporating natural remedies with your doctor to determine if they are appropriate for your case. Use them properly and safely.

Soothing Teas and Herbs that Can Help Manage Acid Reflux Symptoms

Certain herbal teas and medicinal herbs have properties that help calm an upset stomach, reduce inflammation, and ease acid reflux discomfort. Sipping tea and taking herbs under the guidance of your doctor can aid in managing symptoms naturally.

1. **Ginger tea:** Ginger root soothes the gastrointestinal tract and reduces spasms, gas, nausea, and cramping. Steep sliced fresh ginger or use tea bags as needed for reflux relief.
2. **Chamomile tea:** Chamomile is an effective anti-inflammatory agent that can soothe an inflamed esophagus caused by stomach acid irritation. Avoid it for those allergic to ragweed.
3. **Peppermint tea:** Peppermint reduces muscle spasms and relaxes the lower esophageal sphincter

when reflux flares up. Do not drink daily, as it may exacerbate symptoms long-term.

4. **Marshmallow root tea:** The mucilage from marshmallow root coats and protects mucus membranes in the throat and esophagus from acid burn.

5. **Fennel tea:** Fennel is known to relax intestinal muscles and soothe digestive upset, with its anise flavor bringing added comfort to post-meal reflux symptoms.

6. **Slippery elm:** Another demulcent herb, slippery elm bark, contains mucilage that lines and shields the esophagus from acid erosion. Available in lozenges.

7. **Licorice root:** Licorice increases protective mucus production in the stomach. However, limit intake due to potential side effects like high blood pressure.

8. **DGL supplements:** Deglycyrrhizinated licorice (DGL) supplements provide healing benefits for the esophagus without the risks of whole licorice.

Always select high-quality herbs from reputable suppliers. Discuss proper dosing and contraindications with your doctor before use, especially if taking other medications or supplements. Herbal remedies nicely complement lifestyle changes.

Recommended Supplements That Can Help Manage Acid Reflux

In addition to diet and lifestyle measures, certain nutritional supplements can support digestive health and help prevent acid reflux symptoms. Some key supplements to consider include:

1. **Probiotics:** Probiotic supplements replenish healthy gut bacteria to optimize digestion and reduce inflammation. Look for multi-strain formulas with billions of CFUs from brands like Align, Culturelle, or Renew Life.

2. **Digestive enzymes:** Enzymes like amylase, lipase, and protease bolster the chemical breakdown of foods, easing the digestive workload. This prevents undigested food from causing excess pressure on the LES.

3. **Zinc carnosine:** Zinc repairs damaged esophageal tissues and stimulates protective compounds. Multiple studies demonstrate zinc carnosine's benefits for healing ulcers and erosions and reducing acid reflux.

4. **DGL licorice:** DGL (deglycyrrhizinated licorice) supplements increase protective mucus production in the stomach without the potential side effects of whole licorice root.

5. **Melatonin:** A study found melatonin significantly decreased GERD symptoms and esophageal damage by strengthening the lower esophageal sphincter and normalizing gastric secretions.

6. **Gamma-oryzanol:** This antioxidant compound derived from rice bran oil improved reflux symptoms in several trials. It reduces inflammation and stomach acid secretion.

Be sure to consult a physician before taking supplements, especially if you take other medications or have a medical condition. While generally well tolerated, some supplements may interact with medications or exacerbate certain health problems. Follow the dosing recommendations carefully.

Supplements work best alongside the dietary and lifestyle changes detailed in this book. A multifaceted, natural approach addresses the root causes of acid reflux for lasting relief. With your doctor's guidance, supplements can enhance prevention efforts.

Breathing Exercises and Stress Reduction Techniques

Stress significantly exacerbates acid reflux symptoms. Breathing deeply and employing relaxation techniques can relieve flare-ups and reduce episodes overall.

Deep, diaphragmatic breathing maximizes the oxygenation needed for proper digestion. Place one hand on your chest and the other on your belly. Inhale slowly through your nose, feeling your abdomen expand with breath. Exhale fully, focusing on long, slow, controlled breaths. Practice for 5–10 minutes daily.

Meditation and mindfulness quell stress hormones that trigger acid production and relax the LES. Try a 15-minute guided meditation app session morning and night. Focus on your breathing while letting distracting thoughts float away.

Yoga incorporates breathwork, mindfulness, and stretches to induce full-body relaxation—gentle poses, like the child's pose, massage the internal organs. Inversions, like legs up the wall, allow gravity to aid digestion.

Listen to soothing music or nature sounds while visualizing a peaceful scene. Music therapy lowers anxiety markers like heart rate and blood pressure.

Unplug from digital devices and screens for a set time before bed. The blue light stimulates brain activity, making it harder to wind down. Read an uplifting book instead.

Spend time outdoors walking or gardening. Fresh air and vitamin D production reduce stress. Choose relaxing hobbies like painting, crafting, or journaling.

Talk to a close friend or journal your thoughts and worries. Do not bottle up emotions; healthily express them.

Learn your personal stress triggers and plan healthy responses. Maintain realistic expectations for yourself. Say no to added obligations.

Try natural supplements like magnesium, omega-3s, or adaptogens to enhance resilience. Consult your doctor first regarding safety and potential interactions.

With practice, stress management becomes a healthy habit. By learning to relax both body and mind, you will minimize a major trigger of acid reflux flare-ups.

Chapter 4

Medications and Medical Procedures

Common Medical Treatment Options for Acid Reflux and GERD

If symptoms persist despite lifestyle modifications, several classes of medications can provide relief from reflux. Common prescription drugs include:

1. **Antacids:** These over-the-counter medications provide rapid but short-term symptom relief by neutralizing stomach acid. Brands include Tums, Rolaids, and Maalox.

2. **H2 receptor blockers:** Medications like cimetidine (Tagamet) and famotidine (Pepcid) reduce acid

production by blocking histamine receptors. It is used to heal mild esophagitis.

3. **Proton pump inhibitors:** Omeprazole (Prilosec), lansoprazole (Prevacid), and other PPIs more potently block acid production and are used for more severe, chronic GERD cases.

4. **Prokinetics:** These medications aid digestion by strengthening the lower esophageal sphincter and promoting stomach emptying. Examples are metoclopramide (Reglan) and domperidone (Motilium).

5. **Sucralfate:** Sucralfate coats and protects damaged esophageal tissue while suppressing acid production. Reduces heartburn pain and helps heal ulcers.

In addition to medications, certain medical procedures can provide relief for those with chronic, unresponsive GERD:

1. **Fundoplication surgery:** This procedure wraps and tightens the upper portion of the stomach around the lower esophageal sphincter to strengthen it and prevent reflux.

2. **LINX device:** A magnetic bracelet implanted laparoscopically around the LES reinforces the valve, allowing food and liquid to pass normally.

3. **Stretta procedure:** Using a catheter, radiofrequency energy thickens and strengthens esophageal tissues just above the LES.

Discuss the benefits and risks of medications versus procedures with your doctor to determine the most appropriate options based on your case. The right treatment brings sustained relief and improves quality of life.

Pros and Cons of Using Common Acid Reflux Medications

Antacids	
Pros:	**Cons:**
Provide rapid relief for mild, intermittent symptoms.	Effects only last 1-2 hours.
Inexpensive and available over-the-counter.	Large doses can cause diarrhea or constipation.
Very safe for short-term use.	It may impact the absorption of other medications and nutrients.
	Not a solution for chronic GERD.

H2 Blockers (Tagamet, Pepcid, etc.)	
Pros:	**Cons:**
Stronger acid reduction than antacids.	It may take several days to start providing symptom relief.
Heal mild esophagitis by allowing damaged tissues to recover.	Efficacy decreases with prolonged use as the body adapts.
Less costly than proton pump inhibitors.	It is not as potent for serious, chronic GERD.
	Can interfere with nutrient absorption.

Proton Pump Inhibitors (Prilosec, Prevacid, etc.)	
Pros:	**Cons:**
The most potent acid reduction available.	The most expensive class of reflux medications.
Heal severe inflammation and erosions.	There are higher risks of side effects like diarrhea, headaches, and nausea.
Prevent complications from uncontrolled GERD.	Decreases absorption of vitamin B12, calcium, iron, and magnesium.
	It should not be used long-term or unnecessarily.

While drugs can manage symptoms, they do not address the underlying causes of reflux. Lifestyle changes should be exhausted first. Use medications only as needed, in consultation with your physician, to supplement prevention strategies.

Surgical Procedures to Treat Severe, Chronic Acid Reflux

For those with intractable GERD symptoms that persist despite maximal medical therapy, surgical intervention may be warranted. Fundoplication surgery is the most common procedure performed for severe gastroesophageal reflux disease.

During the laparoscopic operation, the upper portion of the stomach is wrapped around the lower esophageal sphincter and sutured into place. This reinforces the LES valve mechanism by increasing pressure at the junction of the esophagus and stomach. The wrapped portion prevents the backflow of stomach contents into the esophagus.

Fundoplication surgery achieves several beneficial effects for chronic reflux:

- It tightens and strengthens the malfunctioning lower esophageal sphincter.

- Increases intra-abdominal pressure to prevent reflux
- Reduces hiatal hernia size
- Limits the ability of air or liquid to reflux upwards into the esophagus
- Decreases acid production long-term

Benefits of the surgery include complete or near elimination of GERD symptoms like heartburn, regurgitation, and nausea in about 90% of patients. Many can stop taking reflux medications.

Possible complications include difficulty swallowing, bloating, flatulence, diarrhea, or vomiting if the wrap is too tight. Rarely, the wrap can come undone, requiring additional surgery.

Exhausting all lifestyle modifications and medical management strategies before surgery is critical. However, for those with severe reflux complications or persistent symptoms despite other treatments, fundoplication can be life-changing. Discuss thoroughly with your doctor.

When Conventional Medical Treatment for Acid Reflux May be Necessary.

Lifestyle and dietary changes should always be the first line of defense against acid reflux. However, conventional medications or procedures may become necessary when natural approaches alone are insufficient. Examples include:

- The presence of severe erosions, ulcers, strictures, or Barrett's esophagus was detected on endoscopy. These complications require stronger treatment to enable healing.
- Acid reflux that persists at night despite head elevation, sleeping on the left side, and avoidance of food 3 hours before bed. Nighttime symptoms disrupt sleep and impair the quality of life.
- Dietary and lifestyle modifications are insufficient to alleviate chronic hoarseness, sore throat, coughing, or asthma, indicating that more intensive treatment is needed for laryngopharyngeal reflux (LPR).
- Persistent regurgitation of stomach contents into the mouth despite dietary modifications greatly impacts daily functioning and increases aspiration risk.
- Bothersome symptoms that continue despite eliminating trigger foods, losing excess weight, quitting smoking, etc. Severe cases may need stronger acid suppression.

- Frequent use of over-the-counter antacids without lasting relief. H2 blockers or PPIs may better control symptoms long-term.

- Difficulty swallowing indicates a stricture that requires medications or procedures to open the esophagus.

- The presence of a large hiatal hernia does not respond to attempts to reduce pressure on the LES through diet and lifestyle. Surgery may be an option.

- Intolerable, persistent symptoms that significantly undermine the quality of life. Advanced treatments provide an improved quality of life.

Remember, the goal is to use medications and procedures only as needed to supplement natural prevention strategies. Work closely with your doctor to determine your case's most appropriate treatment plan. Many find complete relief through lifestyle adjustments alone when applied diligently.

Chapter 5

Preventing Acid Reflux in Children and Infants

The Common Causes of Acid Reflux in Infants and Children

Acid reflux, also known as gastroesophageal reflux (GER), is common in babies and children. A variety of factors can contribute to reflux in the pediatric population.

In infants, the predominant cause is the immaturity of the lower esophageal sphincter (LES) and digestive system. The sphincter does not close properly, allowing stomach contents to backwash into the esophagus. This muscle strengthens as the child develops.

A common cause of acid reflux in newborns is a hiatal hernia, which occurs when part of the stomach moves up through the diaphragm and affects the LES. This condition often resolves itself within the first year.

Babies also have a liquid-based diet of breast milk or formula. These liquid feeds can easily regurgitate back up when the LES relaxes. Spitting up is normal for many infants after feeding.

Food allergies and sensitivities provoke reflux in some children, especially to proteins in formula or cow's milk. Food intolerances create inflammation and irritate the intestinal lining.

Children's smaller stomachs are more easily overfilled, causing reflux. Overfeeding or forcing children to finish bottles while overriding their fullness cues is problematic. Carbonated beverages and juices further exacerbate reflux.

Obesity and excess weight put pressure on the LES and hiatal canal in overweight children. Carrying extra pounds in the abdomen contributes greatly to pediatric GERD.

Asthma and reflux are interrelated in many children. Acidic reflux can trigger asthma flares, while asthma medications like theophylline relax the LES, promoting reflux.

Thankfully, reflux resolves independently in most babies by 12–24 months as the LES strengthens and the diet solidifies. Simple natural remedies and feeding adjustments typically manage mild cases effectively.

Lifestyle Changes Parents Can Implement to Help Prevent and Manage Acid Reflux in Children

Making lifestyle adjustments can alleviate acid reflux in babies and children without requiring medications in mild cases. Natural prevention strategies for kids include:

1. **Smaller, more frequent feedings:** Avoid overfilling the stomach by offering smaller portions more often. Slow, paced bottle feeding also helps.

2. **Keeping infants upright during and after feeds:** Hold infants upright for 15–30 minutes following a feeding to allow gravity to aid digestion.

3. **Propping up in bed:** For young children, elevate the head of the bed 4-6 inches to prevent nighttime reflux when lying flat.

4. **Avoiding food triggers:** Dairy, soy, citrus, and acidic foods provoke symptoms in some children. Identify the problem foods.

5. **Encouraging active play:** Exercise improves digestion and prevents obesity. Outdoor play also exposes kids to vitamin D from sunlight.

6. **Dressing in loose clothing:** Tight clothes add pressure to the abdomen, worsening reflux. Choose soft, breathable fabrics.

7. **Probiotic foods and supplements:** Probiotics like yogurt improve gut health and digestion to reduce reflux. Consult your pediatrician first.

8. **Soothing teas:** Ginger, fennel, or chamomile tea may safely ease occasional reflux discomfort. Ask your pediatrician.

9. **Managing stress and encouraging rest:** Stress exacerbates reflux. Make sure children get naps and quiet time.

10. **Quitting secondhand smoke exposure:** If parents smoke, take it outside and away from children. Secondhand smoke irritates the reflux.

11. **Monitoring weight:** Carrying excess weight strains the LES. Ensure proper nutrition and exercise.

Simple adjustments tailored to your child often successfully relieve mild reflux. If symptoms persist or seem severe, consult your pediatrician and pediatric gastroenterologist.

Safe and Effective Natural Remedies to Relieve Acid Reflux in Infants and Children

Several natural solutions can safely provide symptomatic relief when babies and kids experience acid reflux flare-ups. Always consult your pediatrician before administering any remedies to ensure their appropriateness for your child. Helpful options include:

1. **Gripe water:** Over-the-counter gripe water contains herbs like fennel and ginger to ease colic and mild reflux discomfort in infants. Give 1-3 mL as needed.

2. **Chamomile tea:** The anti-inflammatory properties of chamomile tea may reduce reflux swelling and irritation when cooled and given in small amounts to children over 6 months old.

3. **Slippery elm:** As a thickening demulcent, slippery elm coats and protects the esophageal lining from acid irritation when mixed with water or juice.

4. **Probiotic drops:** Probiotic drops promote healthy gut flora and digestion. Choose infant-specific brands with limited strains. Give per-label instructions.

5. **Rice cereal:** Consult with your pediatrician before adding a spoon or two of rice cereal to bottles. It can thicken the feed and reduce reflux.

6. **Skin-to-skin contact:** Infant skin-to-skin contact provides comfort and facilitates burping and digestion.

7. **Honey sticks:** For children over 1, honey sticks provide immediate symptom relief and coat the throat. Use sparingly due to the botulism risk.

8. **Diet changes:** If reflux correlates with certain foods, try eliminating dairy, soy, wheat, and acidic foods. Reintroduce one at a time.

9. **Gas drops:** Over-the-counter simethicone drops like Mylicon can help relieve painful gas bubbles. Always follow age guidelines.

10. **Cool liquids:** Clear liquids like water or aloe vera juice may coat and soothe irritated tissues. Do not give honey.

Monitor your child closely and avoid any remedy that seems to worsen symptoms or cause side effects. Natural remedies work best alongside feeding adjustments and lifestyle changes.

When to See a Pediatrician Regarding Acid Reflux Symptoms in Babies and Children

Frequent regurgitation and spitting up are common in many healthy infants. However, severe or persistent reflux symptoms in babies and children may warrant medical evaluation. See a pediatrician promptly if your child experiences:

- Projectile vomiting or forceful spitting up consistently after feeding
- Vomit that is green or yellow, bloody, or smells bad
- Unexplained crying fits, irritability, or discomfort during or after feeding
- Inconsolable crying for over 3 hours daily
- Refusing to eat, having difficulty swallowing, or gagging during feeds
- Poor weight gain or failure to gain weight appropriately
- Spitting up more than 4 times per day after being 6 months old
- Frequent coughing, wheezing, or breathlessness
- Hoarse crying, chronic sore throat, or cough
- Recurrent lung infections or pneumonia
- Tooth enamel erosion or decay

These signs may indicate a more serious condition, like pyloric stenosis, a milk protein allergy, or chronic respiratory issues aggravated by reflux. Severe vomiting can also cause dangerous weight loss or dehydration.

Seek emergency care for any breathing struggles, blue coloration of skin, legs, or lips, or choking during feeds. This may signal a blocked airway.

Call your pediatrician if over-the-counter antacids or lifestyle changes do not relieve symptoms in 2 weeks. Chronic acid reflux may require prescription medication or testing for underlying causes.

Do not hesitate to have your child evaluated, even if the symptoms seem mild. The pediatrician can help determine if further treatment is needed or reassure that things are progressing normally.

Conclusion

Acid reflux, or gastroesophageal reflux disease (GERD), affects millions of adults and children worldwide. While incredibly common, chronic reflux severely impacts the quality of life if left unchecked. The great news is that simple diet and lifestyle changes can often prevent symptoms without relying on medications.

This comprehensive guide outlined the physiology behind reflux and identified the risk factors that provoke it. We can target lifestyle habits by understanding what causes the lower esophageal sphincter to malfunction—losing excess weight, avoiding trigger foods, managing stress, elevating the head at night, and wearing loose clothing all control reflux.

Implementing a GERD-friendly diet is critical. We discussed the many delicious, nourishing foods that are safe to eat freely and the acidic, fat-laden options to limit. Smaller, more balanced meals are vital as well. Natural remedies like aloe, licorice, and slippery elm soothe flare-ups when they strike. Probiotics, DGL, and select supplements further boost your defenses.

For chronic sufferers, a step-down approach to antacids paired with prevention techniques provides true relief without permanent reliance on medications with side effects. Based on the severity, we reviewed cases where medical treatment may still be warranted. However, for most, the holistic toolkit equips you to prevent acid reflux successfully and permanently.

Consistency is key in managing GERD through diet and lifestyle changes. Simply making sporadic adjustments or trying out a few remedies will not solve the problem. In order to experience lasting freedom from GERD, it is important to diligently follow a full program that includes changes in diet, stress relief, sleep positioning, smaller meals, trigger avoidance, and natural remedies. By doing so, you can take control of your life and significantly improve your quality of life.

The Comprehensive Plan to Prevent and Manage Acid Reflux Naturally

This comprehensive guide provides a complete acid reflux management plan that includes:

- Dietary modifications like avoiding trigger foods, smaller or lighter meals, remaining upright after eating, sufficient chewing, and proper hydration
- Lifestyle adjustments, including losing excess weight if your BMI is over 25, wearing loose clothing, quitting smoking, limiting alcohol, and stress management
- Proper sleep positioning involves elevating the head 4–8 inches and avoiding eating within 3 hours of bedtime.
- Natural remedies and soothing foods like aloe, licorice, baking soda, ginger, chamomile, apples, and green vegetables
- Helpful supplements such as zinc, carnosine, DGL, probiotics, and melatonin should be taken under a doctor's supervision.
- Breathing exercises, meditation, yoga, music therapy, and other relaxation techniques

- Weaning off dependence on antacids and acid blockers by gradually stepping down usage while applying lifestyle changes
- Recognizing warning signs indicating when conventional treatment may be necessary for severe, persistent reflux
- Preventative measures tailored for babies and children, like more frequent, smaller feeds, keeping infants upright during and after feeding, probiotics, gripe water, and rice cereal in bottles

The key is consistency in implementing the full range of dietary, lifestyle, and behavioral changes that impact acid reflux. Employing natural preventative measures diligently without relying solely on antacids empowers you to achieve freedom from reflux for good.

With the comprehensive guidance in this book, you can break your dependence on medications and experience excellent health by putting proven acid reflux management techniques into daily practice. Long-term relief is within your grasp!

The Importance of Consistency and Patience When Applying Natural Acid Reflux Management Techniques

Implementing this book's comprehensive LIFESTYLE and dietary modifications is life-changing for acid reflux sufferers. However, real results require commitment, consistency, and patience. Quick fixes and sporadic changes will not lead to lasting relief.

Understand that the damage from chronic acid reflux develops over months or years. Healing and strengthening the esophagus happen gradually as well. Allow at least 2–3 months of diligent adherence to your customized management plan to fully resolve symptoms.

Attempting too many changes simultaneously can lead to poor compliance. Introduce new diet and lifestyle measures gradually over several weeks to make them stick. Small steps add up to big results.

There will inevitably be setbacks and slip-ups, especially with trigger foods or heavy meals. Do not let perfectionism lead to abandoning your plan. Just get back on track at the next meal or day. Progress, not perfection, is key.

Keep tweaking your individual prevention plan based on your body's signals until you find the specific changes that provide relief for you. For example, elevating your upper body 6 inches at night may ease symptoms better than 4 inches.

Track symptoms and correlate them to potential triggers or slip-ups in your management plan. This helps identify problematic areas to refine. Communication with your doctor ensures proper progress.

With regular adherence to the strategies in this book over 2-3 months, most find complete freedom from dependence on antacids and the distress of acid reflux flare-ups. However, commitment and consistency are crucial to experiencing the full benefits.

Take it one day and one positive change at a time. You have all the tools necessary to prevent acid reflux and dramatically improve digestion successfully; now, put them into action with dedication and patience!

Appendices

Weekly Meal Plan with Recipes

Planning healthy, anti-reflux meals is made easy with these delicious sample recipes to enjoy:

Breakfast:	Oatmeal with bananas and slivered almonds
	Veggie and egg white omelet with avocado toast
	Greek yogurt-berry parfait
Lunch:	Turkey and avocado sandwich on sourdough bread
	Lentil vegetable soup with a side salad
	Quinoa tabbouleh stuffed in a pita
Dinner:	Baked salmon with roasted potatoes and Brussels sprouts
	Chicken stir-fry with brown rice and broccoli

	Black bean enchilada-stuffed peppers
Snacks:	A small handful of walnuts and grapes
	Carrots and cucumbers with hummus
	Apple slices with sunflower seed butter
Beverages:	Herbal teas like chamomile, ginger, or licorice
	Low-acid fruit smoothies with plant milk
	Aloe vera or coconut water
Desserts:	Greek yogurt parfait with berry compote
	70% dark chocolate squares
	Rice pudding

Following an eating plan tailored to your reflux triggers ensures you stay symptom-free while enjoying nourishing whole foods. Meal prep and planning ahead are key to making this a sustainable lifestyle.

Shopping Lists

Filling your kitchen with plenty of delicious, low-reflux foods ensures you can create varied, enjoyable meals easily.

Proteins:	• Boneless, skinless chicken and turkey breast • Lean ground turkey or grass-fed beef • Wild-caught fish like salmon, cod, and tuna • Eggs, preferably free-range • Plant-based proteins like tofu, tempeh, lentils, and black beans
Grains:	• Old-fashioned oats, gluten-free oats • Brown rice, quinoa, and buckwheat • Sourdough or whole-grain bread
Fruits:	• Bananas, melons, apples, grapes, and berries • Unsweetened applesauce • Avocado
Vegetables:	• Cruciferous veggies: broccoli, Brussels sprouts, cabbage • Root vegetables like potatoes, carrots, and beets • Leafy greens: spinach, kale, lettuce, and Swiss chard

	• Zucchini, green beans, asparagus, and celery
Dairy:	• Low-fat plain Greek yogurt • Plant-based milk like almond, oat, or coconut • Non-dairy cheese like Daiya
Beverages:	• Herbal tea: chamomile, ginger, licorice, and fennel • Coconut water • Low-acid vegetable and fruit juices

Stocking your kitchen allows you to whip up reflux-friendly meals with ease. Meal prep staples like bone broth, quinoa, whole grain bread, and roasted veggies are great to have on hand.

Recipes for Reflux-Friendly Meals

It is possible to enjoy delicious meals while following an acid-reflux diet. These recipes make it easy to eat well and feel good.

Chili-Lime Chicken Bowls

<u>Ingredients:</u>

- 2 boneless, skinless chicken breasts, pounded to 1/2 inch thickness
- 2 tablespoons extra virgin olive oil
- 3 cloves garlic, minced
- 1 jalapeno, seeded and diced
- Juice from 1 lime
- 1 15-ounce can of black beans, drained and rinsed
- 1 cup of cooked brown rice
- 2 cups baby spinach
- 1 avocado, sliced
- Fresh cilantro for garnish

<u>Instructions:</u>

1. Season the chicken with salt, pepper, chili powder, and a pinch of cayenne. Heat 1 tablespoon of oil in a skillet over medium-high heat. Cook the chicken

for 5 minutes per side until browned and cooked through. Let it rest for 5 minutes before slicing.

2. Heat the remaining 1 tablespoon of oil in a skillet. Add garlic and jalapeno, cooking for 1 minute. Add beans and spinach; cook until wilted, about 2 minutes.

3. Serve the chicken over the rice and bean mixture. Top with avocado slices, lime juice, and cilantro.

Vegan Minestrone Soup

Ingredients:
- 2 Tbsp. olive oil
- 1 onion, diced
- 3 carrots, sliced
- 3 stalks of celery, chopped
- 1 zucchini, quartered and sliced
- 6 cups of vegetable broth
- 1 (14.5 oz) can diced tomatoes
- 1 (15-ounce) can of white beans, drained and rinsed
- 2 cups of packed baby spinach
- 2 Tbsp. basil pesto
- 1 tsp. oregano
- Red pepper flakes, to taste

Instructions:

1. Heat oil in a large pot over medium heat. Add the onion, carrots, and celery. Cook for 5 minutes.
2. Add zucchini, broth, tomatoes, beans, spinach, and seasonings. Bring to a boil.
3. Reduce heat and simmer for 10 minutes until veggies are tender.
4. Remove from heat and stir in basil pesto.
5. Serve with whole-grain bread, if desired. Sprinkle with red pepper flakes.

Baked Salmon with Garlic Broccoli

Ingredients:

- 4 (6 oz) salmon fillets
- 2 tbsp. olive oil
- 3 cloves garlic, minced
- 1 lb. broccoli florets
- Lemon wedges

Instructions:

1. Preheat the oven to 400°F. Line a baking sheet with parchment paper.
2. Place the salmon fillets on the prepared baking sheet. Brush the tops with olive oil and season with salt and pepper.

3. Roast the salmon for 12–15 minutes until it is opaque and flakes easily.

4. Meanwhile, toss broccoli florets with minced garlic and 1 tablespoon olive oil. Roast broccoli alongside salmon for 10–12 minutes until tender.

5. Serve salmon over broccoli, squeezing fresh lemon juice over the top.

Chicken and Quinoa Salad

Ingredients:

- 1 lb. boneless, skinless chicken breasts, cooked and diced
- 1 cup of cooked quinoa
- 1 avocado, diced
- 1 cup cherry tomatoes, halved
- 1/4 cup fresh basil, sliced
- 2 tbsp. olive oil
- 2 tbsp. red wine vinegar
- Salt and pepper to taste

Instructions:

1. In a large bowl, combine cooked chicken, quinoa, avocado, tomatoes, and basil.

2. In a small bowl, whisk together olive oil, vinegar, salt, and pepper.

3. Pour the dressing over the salad and toss gently to coat.

Enjoy these anti-reflux recipes as part of a balanced diet tailored to your specific triggers!

References to Research Studies Supporting the Use of Natural Remedies for Acid Reflux

Several clinical studies support the natural acid reflux remedies recommended in this book. Always consult your physician before trying supplements. Here are some key studies:

- **Chewing gum:** Multiple studies have found that chewing gum post-meals stimulates saliva production, clearing acid more quickly. Gum also facilitates swallowing. [1]
- **Aloe vera:** A 2007 trial found oral aloe vera juice significantly reduced heartburn severity and improved quality of life in GERD patients. [2]
- **Slippery elm:** Research indicates slippery elm stimulates mucus production, coats the gastrointestinal lining, and reduces stomach acidity. [3]

- **Zinc carnosine:** Multiple human and animal studies demonstrate that zinc carnosine promotes esophageal healing by enhancing protective factors. [4]

- **Melatonin:** A 2013 study reported that melatonin decreased GERD symptoms by 65% and improved esophageal health by strengthening the LES. [5]

- **DGL licorice:** Deglycyrrhizinated licorice (DGL) has been shown in studies to heal stomach ulcers and improve GERD symptoms. [6]

- **Probiotics:** Specific probiotic strains like Lactobacillus reuteri are documented to reduce reflux events, heal damaged tissue, and boost gastric defenses. [7]

- **Diet:** Research confirms obesity, large meal sizes, high-fat foods, alcohol, chocolate, and smoking increase reflux and esophageal damage. [8]

- **Head elevation:** Elevating the head in bed is proven to reduce nighttime acid reflux events and esophageal acid exposure significantly. [9]

- **Stress management:** Meditation and yoga reduce stress hormone production that drives acid secretion and LES relaxation. [10]

Commitment to the comprehensive lifestyle and diet modifications in this guide allows you to break free from medications and experience excellent digestion. The natural recommendations are evidence-based.

Resources for Finding Support and Community as You Manage Acid Reflux

Implementing major diet and lifestyle changes to overcome acid reflux can feel challenging at times. Connecting with others on a similar journey provides invaluable support and motivation. Here are great resources:

- Join an online acid reflux support group through platforms like Facebook Groups and Inspire. Share tips, recipes, and encouragement with those who understand the daily struggles.
- Connect with an acid reflux coach for expert guidance tailored to your symptoms and triggers. A coach motivates you to stick to your treatment plan and helps problem-solve issues via phone, text, or email.
- The International Foundation for Gastrointestinal Disorders (IFFGD) has a network of support groups you can join to connect with others with GI

conditions in your local area. Meet regularly for sharing and learning.

- Seek out friends and family who will cheer you on and hold you accountable as you implement lifestyle changes. Share your meal plan and triggers to avoid so loved ones can support your new habits.
- Schedule visits with a registered dietitian who specializes in GERD to review your diet overhaul, create meal plans, and suggest reflux-friendly recipes. A dietitian provides professional guidance.
- Consult a psychologist to develop stress-coping techniques. A psychologist can teach you stress management strategies and help you overcome the emotional toll of chronic acid reflux.
- Join cooking classes that focus on anti-reflux recipes. You will discover new delicious, GERD-friendly meals while connecting over a common interest.

With determination and the right support system, you can break free of acid reflux for good. Do not go it alone; tap into the many avenues of understanding and encouragement available to optimize your success. Managing reflux is achievable when you have the right team behind you.